EMPOWER HER

A PCOS WELLNESS GUIDE

By

Dr Lisa Moran

Empower Her: A Pcos Wellness Guide

Copyright @2024 Lisa Moran

All right reserved

Empower Her: A Pcos Wellness Guide

TABLE OF CONTENTS

TABLE OF CONTENTS
Chapter 1
Introduction
   1.1 Definition and Overview of PCOS
   1.2 Significance and Impact on Women's Health
   1.3 Unveiling the Complexity: Anatomy and Physiology
   1.4 Historical Perspective: Stein-Leventhal Syndrome to Modern Recognition
Chapter 2
Understanding PCOS
   2.1 Anatomy and Physiology of the Ovaries
   2.2 Hormonal Imbalances in PCOS
   2.3 Genetic and Environmental Factors
Chapter 3
Epidemiology and Demographics
   3.1 Global Prevalence
   3.2 Ethnic and Age-Related Variances
   3.3 Incidence Rates
   3.4 Impact on Reproductive Health
   3.5 Metabolic Implications and Cardiovascular Risks
   3.6 Challenges in Diagnosis and Misconceptions

Chapter 4
Diagnostic Criteria
- 4.1 National Institutes of Health (NIH) Criteria
- 4.2 Rotterdam Criteria
- 4.3 Challenges in Diagnosis and Misconceptions
- 4.4 Emerging Perspectives on Diagnosis
- 4.5 Diagnostic Tools and Imaging Studies
- 4.6 The Role of Menstrual Health

Chapter 5
Treatment Options for Polycystic Ovary Syndrome (PCOS)
- 5.1 Lifestyle Modifications
  - 5.1.1 Diet and Nutrition
  - 5.1.2 Exercise and Physical Activity
  - 5.1.3 Stress Management
- 5.2 Medications
  - 5.2.1 Oral Contraceptives
  - 5.2.2 Anti-androgen Medications
  - 5.2.3 Insulin-sensitizing Agents
- 5.3 Assisted Reproductive Technologies (ART)
- 5.4 Surgical Interventions

Chapter 6
Managing PCOS-related Complications
- 6.1 Infertility and Fertility Treatments
  - 6.1.1 Understanding Infertility in PCOS
  - 6.1.2 Fertility Treatments: A Multifaceted Approach
  - 6.1.3 Lifestyle Modifications for Fertility
- 6.2 Metabolic and Cardiovascular Risks
  - 6.2.1 Insulin Resistance and Metabolic Syndrome

6.2.2 Cardiovascular Disease in Women with PCOS
6.3 Psychological Impact and Mental Health
6.3.1 Recognizing the Psychological Burden
6.3.2 Coping Strategies and Support
6.4 Integrating Treatment Approaches

Chapter 7
PCOS and Other Health Conditions
7.1 Association with Type 2 Diabetes
7.1.1 The Interplay of Insulin Resistance
7.1.2 Lifestyle Interventions for Diabetes Prevention
7.2 Cardiovascular Disease Risk
7.2.1 Understanding Cardiovascular Risks in PCOS
7.2.2 Lifestyle Modifications for Cardiovascular Health
7.3 Endometrial Cancer Risk
7.3.1 Unraveling the Endometrial Cancer Connection
7.3.2 Preventive Strategies and Surveillance
7.4 Holistic Approaches to Multifaceted Health
7.5 Future Directions in Research and Care
8.1 Nutrition Plans
8.1.1 The Impact of Diet on PCOS Symptoms
8.1.2 Designing a PCOS-Friendly Diet
8.1.3 Nutritional Support for Hormonal Balance
8.2 Exercise Routines
8.2.1 The Role of Exercise in PCOS Management
8.2.2 Developing a Personalized Exercise

Empower Her: A Pcos Wellness Guide

Plan
8.2.3 Overcoming Barriers to Physical Activity
8.3 Weight Management Strategies
8.3.1 The Interconnection of Weight and PCOS
8.3.2 Nutrition and Exercise in Weight Management
8.3.3 Psychological Aspects of Weight Management
8.4 Holistic Lifestyle Integration
8.4.1 Balancing Nutrition, Exercise, and Mental Well-being
8.5 Resources and Support

Chapter 9
Support and Resources for PCOS
9.1 Support Groups
9.1.1 Understanding the Power of Peer Support
9.1.2 Joining Local and Online Support Groups
9.1.3 Support for Specific PCOS Phenotypes
9.2 Educational Materials
9.2.1 Empowering Through Knowledge
9.2.2 Recommended Reading and Resources
9.3 Online Communities
9.3.1 Connecting Virtually
9.3.2 Navigating Online Communities Safely
9.4 Healthcare Professionals
9.4.1 Building a Collaborative Relationship
9.4.2 Choosing the Right Healthcare Team
9.5 Advocacy and Awareness

9.5.1 Empowering Through Advocacy
9.5.2 Participating in Awareness Campaigns
9.6 Coping Strategies and Self-Care
    9.6.1 Nurturing Mental and Emotional Well-being
9.6.2 Balancing Self-Care with Advocacy
9.7 Building Resilience for the PCOS Journey
9.7.1 Embracing Resilience

Chapter 10
Future Directions in PCOS Research

10.1 Ongoing Studies
10.1.1 Investigating Genetic and Environmental Factors
10.1.2 Longitudinal Studies on PCOS Phenotypes
10.2 Potential Breakthroughs
10.2.1 Advancements in Hormonal Therapies
10.2.2 Personalized Medicine and Treatment Plans
10.3 Lifestyle Interventions and Digital Health
10.3.1 Integrating Technology for Lifestyle Management
    10.3.2 Virtual Health Coaching and Telemedicine
10.4 Fertility Advancements
10.4.1 Innovations in Assisted Reproductive Technologies
10.4.2 Preservation of Ovarian Function
10.5 Addressing Metabolic and Cardiovascular Risks
    10.5.1 Targeting Insulin Resistance with Precision
10.5.2 Cardiovascular Risk Prediction Models

10.6 Psychosocial and Mental Health Considerations
10.6.1 Integrating Mental Health Support
    10.6.2 Online Mental Health Platforms
10.7 Patient-Researcher Collaboration
10.7.1 Shaping Research Priorities Together
10.7.2 Citizen Science Initiatives
10.8 Ethical Considerations and Future Challenges
10.8.1 Ethical Dimensions of PCOS Research
10.8.2 Overcoming Research Gaps and Disparities
10.9 Shaping the Future of PCOS Care
10.9.1 From Bench to Bedside
10.9.2 Empowering Individuals Through Research

Chapter 11

Conclusion - Empowering Individuals with PCOS
11.1 Recapitulation of Key Points
11.2 Empowering Individuals with PCOS
11.2.1 Knowledge as a Catalyst for Self-Advocacy
11.2.2 Navigating Lifestyle Changes with Confidence
11.2.3 Building a Support Network
11.2.4 Collaborating with Healthcare Professionals
11.2.5 Balancing Self-Care with Advocacy
11.3 Future Perspectives in PCOS Care
11.3.1 Patient-Researcher Collaboration
13.3.2 Ethical Considerations and Inclusivity
11.3.3 Bridging the Gap between Research

Empower Her: A Pcos Wellness Guide

<u>and Clinical Practice</u>
<u>Conclusion</u>

CHAPTER 1

INTRODUCTION

1.1 Definition and Overview of PCOS

Polycystic Ovary Syndrome (PCOS) stands as a complex and prevalent endocrine disorder affecting individuals with ovaries. Characterized by a combination of hormonal imbalances, irregular menstrual cycles, and the presence of cysts on the ovaries, PCOS is a condition that warrants attention and understanding. In this introductory chapter, we delve into the fundamental aspects of PCOS, outlining its definition, historical context, and the significance it holds in the realm of women's health.

PCOS, as the name suggests, involves the development of small cysts on the ovaries, contributing to hormonal disturbances and a range of symptoms. The disorder was initially recognized in the early 20th century, with significant contributions from gynecologists Irving F. Stein, Sr.

and Michael L. Leventhal, who published a seminal paper in 1935 highlighting the clinical features of what would later be termed "Stein-Leventhal syndrome."

1.2 Significance and Impact on Women's Health

The significance of PCOS extends beyond its immediate reproductive implications. It is not merely a gynecological concern but a complex metabolic and endocrine disorder with profound effects on a woman's overall health. Understanding PCOS involves recognizing its multifaceted impact, encompassing reproductive health, metabolic well-being, and psychological aspects.

PCOS affects individuals during their reproductive years, typically emerging in adolescence or early adulthood. Its prevalence is noteworthy, with estimates suggesting that it affects approximately 5% to 15% of reproductive-aged women globally. However, these figures are subject to variations based on diagnostic criteria, ethnicity, and geographical location.

As we embark on this journey through the landscape of PCOS, it is crucial to acknowledge the diverse ways in which this syndrome manifests.

PCOS is not a one-size-fits-all condition; rather, it presents itself with a spectrum of symptoms and severity levels. While some may experience irregular menstrual cycles and hirsutism, others may grapple with metabolic disturbances, such as insulin resistance and an increased risk of type 2 diabetes.

The impact of PCOS on fertility cannot be overstated. It is a leading cause of ovulatory infertility, posing challenges for those trying to conceive. Beyond reproduction, PCOS elevates the risk of developing metabolic syndrome and cardiovascular issues, underscoring the need for holistic management and an understanding of the long-term health implications.

1.3 Unveiling the Complexity: Anatomy and Physiology

To comprehend PCOS, one must delve into the intricate anatomy and physiology of the ovaries. The ovaries, essential components of the female reproductive system, house follicles containing eggs. In individuals with PCOS, these follicles do not mature properly, leading to the formation of small, fluid-filled cysts.

Hormonal imbalances play a pivotal role in the manifestation of PCOS symptoms. Elevated levels of androgens, commonly referred to as male hormones, contribute to the development of physical signs such as hirsutism, acne, and male-pattern baldness. Additionally, disruptions in the delicate interplay of hormones like estrogen and progesterone result in irregular menstrual cycles, a hallmark feature of PCOS.

1.4 Historical Perspective: Stein-Leventhal Syndrome to Modern Recognition

The historical trajectory of PCOS unveils a gradual understanding of its clinical features and underlying mechanisms. In the early 20th century, the observations made by Stein and Leventhal marked a pivotal moment in recognizing a distinct syndrome characterized by ovarian dysfunction. However, it took several decades for the medical community to refine the diagnostic criteria and grasp the complexity of PCOS beyond its initial associations with amenorrhea and hirsutism.

In 1990, the National Institutes of Health (NIH) held a conference that established standardized diagnostic criteria for PCOS. This marked a crucial step forward in fostering a unified understanding within the medical community. The criteria encompassed hyperandrogenism, ovulatory dysfunction, and the exclusion of other conditions, laying the groundwork for consistent diagnosis and research.

Further refinement came in 2003 with the introduction of the Rotterdam criteria, which expanded the diagnostic spectrum to include the presence of polycystic ovaries on ultrasound. This broader definition allowed for a more comprehensive understanding of PCOS, recognizing its heterogeneity and diverse presentations.

The historical evolution of PCOS recognition reflects not only advances in medical knowledge but also the ongoing efforts to unravel the complexities of this syndrome. As we navigate through the chapters ahead, it becomes apparent that PCOS is not a static entity but a dynamic condition shaped by genetic predispositions, hormonal dynamics, and environmental influences.

In conclusion, this introductory chapter sets the stage for a comprehensive exploration of PCOS. We have laid the groundwork by defining PCOS, exploring its historical roots, and emphasizing its significance in women's health. As we journey deeper into subsequent chapters, we will unravel the layers of PCOS, from its diagnostic intricacies to the multifaceted impact it exerts on the lives of those affected.

CHAPTER 2

UNDERSTANDING PCOS

2.1 Anatomy and Physiology of the Ovaries

To comprehend Polycystic Ovary Syndrome (PCOS), a foundational understanding of the intricate anatomy and physiology of the ovaries is essential. The ovaries, paired reproductive organs in the female pelvic cavity, play a central role in the menstrual cycle and fertility.

Within the ovaries, thousands of tiny structures called follicles house immature eggs. During each menstrual cycle, a subset of these follicles begins to mature under the influence of hormonal signals. In a healthy cycle, one dominant follicle will release a mature egg during ovulation, marking the midpoint of the menstrual cycle.

In the context of PCOS, this natural process is disrupted. The ovaries of individuals with PCOS often contain numerous small, undeveloped follicles that fail to reach maturity. These underdeveloped follicles accumulate, forming small fluid-filled sacs or cysts. The presence of these cysts contributes to the characteristic appearance of polycystic ovaries observed through ultrasound imaging.

2.2 Hormonal Imbalances in PCOS

PCOS is fundamentally characterized by hormonal imbalances, particularly involving androgens – male hormones that are also present in females, albeit in smaller quantities. Elevated levels of androgens, such as testosterone, contribute to the clinical features associated with PCOS.

The delicate balance of hormones involved in the menstrual cycle is disrupted in individuals with PCOS. Insulin resistance, a common feature of PCOS, further amplifies the hormonal disturbances. Insulin, a hormone responsible for regulating blood sugar levels, becomes less effective in facilitating glucose uptake by cells. As a result, the pancreas produces more insulin, leading to higher circulating levels.

Insulin, in turn, stimulates the ovaries to produce more androgens. This creates a feedback loop, as elevated androgen levels contribute to insulin resistance. The intricate interplay of insulin, androgens, and other hormones creates a hormonal milieu that underlies the varied symptoms of PCOS, including irregular menstrual cycles, hirsutism, and acne.

2.3 Genetic and Environmental Factors

While the exact cause of PCOS remains elusive, both genetic and environmental factors contribute to its development. Research suggests a strong genetic component, with a higher likelihood of PCOS occurring in individuals with a family history of the condition. Specific genetic variants related to insulin signaling, androgen production, and follicle development have been implicated in PCOS susceptibility.

Environmental factors, including lifestyle and exposure to certain conditions during critical developmental periods, also play a role. Obesity, for instance, is associated with an increased risk of PCOS and exacerbates insulin resistance. Conversely, lean individuals can also develop PCOS, indicating the multifaceted nature of its origins.

The interaction between genetic predisposition and environmental influences remains an active area of research. Understanding these factors is crucial for personalized approaches to diagnosis and management, taking into account the unique profile of each individual with PCOS.

As we unravel the complex web of anatomical, physiological, hormonal, and genetic factors contributing to PCOS, it becomes evident that this syndrome is not a simple aberration but a nuanced interplay of various elements. In the subsequent chapters, we will explore how these intricacies manifest in the clinical presentation of PCOS, shedding light on the diverse ways this condition impacts the lives of those affected.

CHAPTER 3

EPIDEMIOLOGY AND DEMOGRAPHICS

3.1 Global Prevalence

Understanding the prevalence of Polycystic Ovary Syndrome (PCOS) is pivotal in addressing its impact on women's health globally. PCOS is recognized as one of the most common endocrine disorders affecting individuals assigned female at birth, with prevalence rates varying across different populations and regions.

Epidemiological studies estimate that PCOS affects approximately 5% to 15% of reproductive-aged women worldwide. However, these figures are subject to variability due to factors such as diagnostic criteria, ethnicity, and geographical location. The heterogeneity of PCOS presentations contributes to challenges in precisely determining its prevalence.

In diverse populations, prevalence rates may differ based on genetic factors and lifestyle patterns. For instance, certain ethnic groups, including South Asian, Mediterranean, and Middle Eastern women, are reported to have higher prevalence rates of PCOS. These variations highlight the importance of considering both genetic and environmental factors when exploring the epidemiology of PCOS.

3.2 Ethnic and Age-Related Variances

PCOS does not manifest uniformly across all ethnic groups. Research suggests that South Asian women, for example, may have a higher prevalence of PCOS compared to other ethnicities. These ethnic variations extend to the clinical presentation of PCOS, with differences in symptom severity and metabolic consequences.

Age is another significant factor influencing the prevalence and diagnosis of PCOS. The syndrome typically emerges during adolescence or early adulthood, and its prevalence tends to decrease with age. The age-related aspect of PCOS is noteworthy, considering that the condition often intersects with reproductive health and fertility concerns.

3.3 Incidence Rates

Incidence rates, indicating the number of new cases of PCOS diagnosed within a specific population over a defined period, contribute to our understanding of the dynamic nature of this syndrome. However, determining precise incidence rates poses challenges due to the gradual onset of PCOS symptoms and variations in diagnostic criteria.

The emergence of PCOS during adolescence or early adulthood influences its incidence rates, as this is a critical period for reproductive and hormonal development. Research into the incidence of PCOS is essential for identifying trends and potential risk factors, facilitating early detection and intervention.

As we explore the global epidemiology of PCOS, it is crucial to recognize the interplay of cultural, genetic, and environmental factors influencing its prevalence. The diversity in PCOS presentations necessitates a nuanced approach to understanding and addressing this complex syndrome on a global scale.

3.4 Impact on Reproductive Health

Beyond the numerical prevalence, the impact of PCOS on reproductive health is a critical facet of its epidemiology. PCOS is a leading cause of ovulatory infertility, contributing to challenges for individuals attempting to conceive. Irregular menstrual cycles, anovulation (lack of ovulation), and other reproductive manifestations of PCOS underscore the significance of this condition in the realm of fertility.

The association between PCOS and fertility complications is multifaceted. While some individuals with PCOS may face challenges in conceiving naturally, others may experience recurrent pregnancy loss or complications during pregnancy. The interplay between hormonal imbalances, disrupted ovulation, and the structural changes in the ovaries contributes to the complexity of PCOS-related infertility.

3.5 Metabolic Implications and Cardiovascular Risks

PCOS is not limited to its reproductive consequences; it extends its influence to metabolic health, elevating the risk of conditions such as insulin resistance, metabolic syndrome, and type 2 diabetes. Understanding the epidemiological link between PCOS and metabolic disorders is crucial for implementing comprehensive healthcare strategies.

Metabolic syndrome, characterized by a cluster of conditions including central obesity, high blood pressure, and abnormal lipid profiles, is more prevalent in individuals with PCOS compared to those without. Insulin resistance, a common feature of PCOS, contributes to the dysregulation of glucose metabolism, increasing the likelihood of developing type 2 diabetes.

Cardiovascular risks also deserve attention in the context of PCOS epidemiology. Individuals with PCOS have an elevated risk of cardiovascular issues, including hypertension and dyslipidemia. The association between PCOS, metabolic syndrome, and cardiovascular risks underscores the need for holistic healthcare approaches that address not only reproductive concerns but also the broader spectrum of health implications.

3.6 Challenges in Diagnosis and Misconceptions

Despite the recognized prevalence of PCOS, challenges in diagnosis persist. The syndrome's diverse clinical presentations, varying symptom severity, and overlapping features with other conditions contribute to diagnostic complexities. Misconceptions surrounding PCOS, such as the notion that it only affects reproductive health or exclusively manifests as ovarian cysts, further complicate accurate and timely diagnosis.

Improving awareness among healthcare professionals and the general public is crucial for overcoming these diagnostic challenges. Enhancing diagnostic precision enables timely intervention and management, reducing the potential long-term health risks associated with PCOS.

In conclusion, this chapter delves into the epidemiology and demographics of PCOS, highlighting its global prevalence, ethnic and age-related variances, and the impact on reproductive and metabolic health. The multifaceted nature of PCOS calls for a nuanced understanding that goes beyond numerical prevalence, acknowledging the complex interplay of factors shaping the epidemiological landscape of this syndrome. As we move forward in this guide, subsequent chapters will explore the diagnostic criteria, clinical manifestations, and management strategies for PCOS, providing a comprehensive approach to this prevalent and impactful condition.

CHAPTER 4

DIAGNOSTIC CRITERIA

4.1 National Institutes of Health (NIH) Criteria

The diagnosis of Polycystic Ovary Syndrome (PCOS) has evolved over the years, with various sets of diagnostic criteria aiming to capture the diverse manifestations of this complex syndrome. Among the earliest and most influential criteria are those established by the National Institutes of Health (NIH).

The NIH criteria, introduced in 1990, provided a standardized framework for diagnosing PCOS. According to these criteria, the diagnosis required the presence of at least two out of three key features:

> Oligo-ovulation or Anovulation: Characterized by irregular menstrual cycles, oligo-ovulation or anovulation refers to infrequent or absent ovulation, a hallmark feature of PCOS.

Clinical or Biochemical Signs of Hyperandrogenism: Elevated levels of androgens, often manifesting as hirsutism (excessive hair growth in typically male-pattern areas), acne, or male-pattern baldness, were considered indicative of PCOS.

Exclusion of Other Conditions: To establish the diagnosis, other conditions with similar clinical features, such as thyroid disorders or hyperprolactinemia, had to be ruled out.

While the NIH criteria provided a valuable framework, they were not without limitations. The emphasis on hyperandrogenism could lead to underdiagnosis in cases where androgen levels were within the normal range, and the criteria did not account for the presence of polycystic ovaries, a common imaging finding in PCOS.

4.2 Rotterdam Criteria

Recognizing the need for a more inclusive and flexible approach to diagnosis, the Rotterdam criteria were introduced in 2003. This consensus-based framework expanded the diagnostic spectrum by including a broader range of features. According to the Rotterdam criteria, a diagnosis of PCOS could be made if two out of three of the following criteria were met:

Oligo-ovulation or Anovulation
Clinical or Biochemical Signs of Hyperandrogenism
Polycystic Ovaries on Ultrasound: Imaging studies revealing the presence of 12 or more follicles in each ovary or an ovarian volume exceeding 10 cm³.

The Rotterdam criteria acknowledged the heterogeneity of PCOS presentations and allowed for a more nuanced diagnosis, incorporating the significance of polycystic ovaries as an additional criterion. However, this inclusivity also posed challenges, as some individuals without hyperandrogenism might be diagnosed based solely on oligo-ovulation and polycystic ovaries.

4.3 Challenges in Diagnosis and Misconceptions

While both the NIH and Rotterdam criteria have been valuable in establishing a standardized approach to PCOS diagnosis, challenges persist. The variability in symptom presentation, the subjective nature of hyperandrogenism assessment, and the potential overlap with other conditions pose diagnostic complexities.

Misconceptions about PCOS further contribute to diagnostic challenges. Some may erroneously believe that the presence of ovarian cysts is a definitive indicator, overlooking the importance of other criteria such as hormonal imbalances and menstrual irregularities. Enhanced awareness among healthcare professionals and the general public is crucial for dispelling these misconceptions and ensuring accurate diagnosis.

Additionally, the evolving understanding of PCOS has prompted ongoing discussions about the need for further refinement of diagnostic criteria. Some experts advocate for a more individualized and tailored approach, considering the diverse phenotypes and presentations observed in PCOS.

4.4 Emerging Perspectives on Diagnosis

As research advances, there is a growing recognition of the need for a comprehensive and personalized approach to PCOS diagnosis. Emerging perspectives emphasize the importance of considering individual symptoms, such as acne or alopecia, as potential indicators of hyperandrogenism. This approach acknowledges the variability in symptom presentation and addresses the limitations of relying solely on traditional signs like hirsutism.

Furthermore, the significance of metabolic features, including insulin resistance and abnormal glucose metabolism, is gaining attention in the diagnostic landscape. Some propose incorporating these metabolic aspects into diagnostic criteria, reflecting the broader impact of PCOS on health beyond the reproductive system.

In the midst of these evolving perspectives, a key challenge is striking the right balance between inclusivity and specificity in diagnostic criteria. The goal is to capture the diverse presentations of PCOS while maintaining the clinical utility and practicality of the diagnostic process.

4.5 Diagnostic Tools and Imaging Studies

Accurate diagnosis often involves a combination of clinical evaluation, blood tests, and imaging studies. Blood tests for hormonal levels, including androgens and reproductive hormones, provide valuable insights into the endocrine profile. However, interpreting these results requires consideration of the menstrual cycle phase and individual variations.

Imaging studies, particularly pelvic ultrasound, play a crucial role in assessing ovarian morphology. The presence of multiple small cysts or follicles in the ovaries, a characteristic finding in PCOS, can be visualized through ultrasound. This imaging modality contributes to the diagnostic process, especially when combined with clinical and hormonal assessments.

4.6 The Role of Menstrual Health

Menstrual health, a central aspect of the diagnostic criteria, reflects the underlying ovulatory dysfunction in PCOS. Irregular menstrual cycles, oligo-ovulation, or anovulation provide critical clues for diagnosis. Tracking menstrual patterns and identifying variations from the norm guide healthcare professionals in evaluating the reproductive aspect of PCOS.

Enhancing the recognition of the importance of menstrual health in PCOS diagnosis is essential. It serves as a window into the hormonal imbalances and ovulatory irregularities characterizing the syndrome. As we delve deeper into the management strategies for PCOS in subsequent chapters, the role of menstrual health remains a focal point for addressing the reproductive challenges associated with this condition.

In conclusion, this chapter explores the diagnostic criteria for PCOS, tracing the historical development from the NIH to the Rotterdam criteria. It highlights the challenges in diagnosis, including misconceptions and the need for ongoing refinement of diagnostic frameworks. The evolving perspectives on PCOS diagnosis emphasize the importance of a personalized and comprehensive approach, acknowledging the diversity of symptoms and phenotypes observed in individuals with PCOS. As we move forward, subsequent chapters will unravel the clinical manifestations, associated health risks, and management strategies for PCOS, providing a holistic understanding of this prevalent and complex syndrome.

CHAPTER 5

TREATMENT OPTIONS FOR POLYCYSTIC OVARY SYNDROME (PCOS)

Polycystic Ovary Syndrome (PCOS) is a complex endocrine disorder that manifests in various ways, affecting the reproductive, metabolic, and psychological aspects of an individual's health. Addressing PCOS requires a comprehensive approach, and Chapter 5 delves into the diverse treatment options available for managing this syndrome.

5.1 Lifestyle Modifications

5.1.1 Diet and Nutrition

One of the primary pillars of PCOS management is adopting a healthy lifestyle, and dietary modifications play a crucial role. Women with PCOS often exhibit insulin resistance, which can be managed through a low-glycemic diet. Chapter 5 explores the benefits of incorporating whole grains, lean proteins, and a variety of fruits and vegetables into the diet. Additionally, the chapter delves into the potential advantages of specific diets, such as the Mediterranean or low-carbohydrate diet, in mitigating PCOS symptoms.

5.1.2 Exercise and Physical Activity

Regular physical activity is another essential aspect of lifestyle modification for women with PCOS. Chapter 5 discusses the positive impact of exercise on insulin sensitivity, weight management, and overall well-being. It provides practical guidance on developing an exercise routine tailored to individual preferences and fitness levels. Whether it's aerobic exercises, strength training, or yoga, the chapter explores the diverse options available and their potential benefits for women with PCOS.

5.1.3 Stress Management

Stress can exacerbate PCOS symptoms, affecting hormonal balance and overall health. In this section, Chapter 5 explores various stress management techniques, including mindfulness meditation, deep breathing exercises, and relaxation strategies. Understanding the interplay between stress and PCOS is crucial for individuals seeking holistic approaches to symptom management.

5.2 Medications

5.2.1 Oral Contraceptives

Oral contraceptives are a common first-line treatment for managing PCOS symptoms. Chapter 5 provides an in-depth analysis of how hormonal contraceptives regulate menstrual cycles, reduce androgen levels, and alleviate symptoms like hirsutism and acne. The chapter also discusses potential side effects and considerations for women with specific health conditions.

5.2.2 Anti-androgen Medications

Certain medications, such as anti-androgens, can help address the elevated levels of androgens associated with PCOS. Spironolactone, for example, is explored in detail in this section, discussing its mechanism of action, potential benefits, and precautions. The chapter emphasizes the importance of individualized treatment plans and close monitoring by healthcare professionals when incorporating anti-androgen medications into the management strategy.

5.2.3 Insulin-sensitizing Agents

Insulin resistance is a common feature of PCOS, and insulin-sensitizing agents like metformin are explored in Chapter 5. The section discusses how these medications improve insulin sensitivity, regulate menstrual cycles, and may contribute to weight management. It also delves into ongoing research on the long-term effects and potential benefits of combining insulin-sensitizing agents with other PCOS treatments.

5.3 Assisted Reproductive Technologies (ART)

For women with PCOS facing infertility, Chapter 5 addresses the role of Assisted Reproductive Technologies (ART). In vitro fertilization (IVF) and other fertility treatments are discussed, highlighting success rates, considerations, and the emotional aspects of fertility interventions. The chapter emphasizes the importance of personalized treatment plans and the involvement of fertility specialists in guiding individuals through the decision-making process.

5.4 Surgical Interventions

In cases where medications and lifestyle modifications may not suffice, surgical interventions become a consideration. Chapter 5 explores procedures such as ovarian drilling, discussing their potential benefits in restoring ovulation and fertility. The section also outlines the risks and considerations associated with surgical interventions, emphasizing the importance of a thorough discussion between patients and healthcare providers.

Chapter 5 provides a comprehensive overview of the diverse treatment options available for managing PCOS. Recognizing the heterogeneity of PCOS presentations, the chapter underscores the importance of individualized treatment plans tailored to address the specific needs and goals of each woman with PCOS. It encourages collaboration between healthcare professionals and individuals affected by PCOS to navigate the complexities of treatment and achieve optimal health outcomes.

CHAPTER 6

MANAGING PCOS-RELATED COMPLICATIONS

Polycystic Ovary Syndrome (PCOS) is a multifaceted condition that extends beyond its immediate reproductive implications, impacting various aspects of a woman's health. Chapter 6 delves into the intricacies of managing PCOS-related complications, addressing challenges such as infertility, metabolic risks, and the psychological impact on overall well-being.

6.1 Infertility and Fertility Treatments

6.1.1 Understanding Infertility in PCOS

Infertility is a prevalent concern for women with PCOS due to irregular ovulation and hormonal imbalances. Chapter 6 initiates the discussion by elucidating the factors contributing to infertility in PCOS, emphasizing the significance of comprehensive fertility assessments. It explores how irregular menstrual cycles and anovulation can impede conception and the emotional toll infertility may take on individuals and couples.

6.1.2 Fertility Treatments: A Multifaceted Approach

This section provides an in-depth exploration of fertility treatments tailored to address PCOS-related infertility. From ovulation-inducing medications like clomiphene citrate to more advanced interventions such as in vitro fertilization (IVF), Chapter 6 offers insights into the effectiveness, risks, and considerations associated with each approach. The chapter underscores the importance of collaboration between reproductive endocrinologists and individuals with PCOS to navigate the intricate journey of fertility treatments.

6.1.3 Lifestyle Modifications for Fertility

In addition to medical interventions, the chapter discusses the role of lifestyle modifications in enhancing fertility. Optimizing body weight through diet and exercise, managing stress, and adopting healthy habits are explored as complementary strategies to improve fertility outcomes. The integration of these lifestyle modifications into a holistic fertility plan is emphasized, acknowledging their potential to positively impact reproductive health.

6.2 Metabolic and Cardiovascular Risks

6.2.1 Insulin Resistance and Metabolic Syndrome

Metabolic disturbances, including insulin resistance, are common in PCOS and contribute to an increased risk of metabolic syndrome. Chapter 6 elucidates the intricate relationship between PCOS, insulin resistance, and metabolic complications such as obesity, type 2 diabetes, and dyslipidemia. The section emphasizes the importance of regular monitoring and early intervention to mitigate long-term metabolic risks.

6.2.2 Cardiovascular Disease in Women with PCOS

Women with PCOS face an elevated risk of cardiovascular diseases. This section explores the underlying mechanisms linking PCOS to cardiovascular risks, emphasizing the role of insulin resistance, inflammation, and hormonal imbalances. Chapter 6 outlines preventive strategies, including lifestyle modifications, cardiovascular screenings, and the management of individual risk factors, to reduce the long-term cardiovascular impact of PCOS.

6.3 Psychological Impact and Mental Health

6.3.1 Recognizing the Psychological Burden

PCOS extends beyond physical symptoms, influencing mental health and well-being. Chapter 6 delves into the psychological impact of PCOS, addressing issues such as anxiety, depression, and body image concerns. It emphasizes the importance of acknowledging and validating the emotional struggles associated with PCOS, fostering a holistic approach to care.

6.3.2 Coping Strategies and Support

This section provides practical insights into coping strategies for individuals grappling with the psychological aspects of PCOS. From psychotherapy and counseling to support groups and online communities, Chapter 6 explores the diverse avenues for emotional support. It underscores the role of healthcare professionals in recognizing and addressing the mental health dimensions of PCOS, promoting a comprehensive approach to care.

6.4 Integrating Treatment Approaches

Recognizing the interconnected nature of PCOS-related complications, Chapter 6 concludes by advocating for an integrated approach to treatment. It emphasizes the importance of collaboration between reproductive endocrinologists, endocrinologists, cardiologists, mental health professionals, and individuals with PCOS to develop personalized treatment plans that address both immediate symptoms and long-term health risks.

The chapter serves as a comprehensive guide for individuals and healthcare providers navigating the intricate landscape of PCOS-related complications. By addressing infertility, metabolic risks, and psychological well-being, Chapter 6 empowers readers to take a proactive role in managing the diverse challenges associated with PCOS. It encourages a holistic perspective that goes beyond symptomatic relief, fostering a comprehensive understanding of PCOS and its impact on women's health across the reproductive, metabolic, and psychological domains.

CHAPTER 7

PCOS AND OTHER HEALTH CONDITIONS

Polycystic Ovary Syndrome (PCOS) is a complex medical condition with far-reaching implications, extending beyond its primary reproductive and endocrine manifestations. Chapter 7 explores the intricate connections between PCOS and other health conditions, shedding light on the associations with Type 2 diabetes, cardiovascular diseases, and the potential risk of endometrial cancer.

7.1 Association with Type 2 Diabetes

7.1.1 The Interplay of Insulin Resistance

Insulin resistance, a hallmark of PCOS, plays a crucial role in the association between PCOS and Type 2 diabetes. Chapter 7 begins by unraveling the mechanisms behind insulin resistance in PCOS and its contribution to glucose dysregulation. It discusses the increased risk of developing Type 2 diabetes in women with PCOS and emphasizes the importance of proactive screening and early intervention to manage and prevent diabetes.

7.1.2 Lifestyle Interventions for Diabetes Prevention

Building upon the theme of lifestyle modifications, this section explores specific strategies to mitigate the risk of Type 2 diabetes in women with PCOS. Dietary interventions, exercise regimens, and weight management are discussed as integral components of a comprehensive approach to reduce insulin resistance and improve glucose metabolism. Chapter 7 highlights the role of healthcare providers in guiding individuals with PCOS toward proactive diabetes prevention strategies.

7.2 Cardiovascular Disease Risk

7.2.1 Understanding Cardiovascular Risks in PCOS

PCOS is associated with an increased risk of cardiovascular diseases, encompassing conditions such as hypertension, dyslipidemia, and atherosclerosis. This section of the chapter delves into the intricate links between hormonal imbalances, insulin resistance, and cardiovascular risks. It emphasizes the need for heightened awareness, early risk assessment, and tailored interventions to address and mitigate the cardiovascular impact of PCOS.

7.2.2 Lifestyle Modifications for Cardiovascular Health

Expanding on lifestyle modifications, Chapter 7 explores how adopting heart-healthy habits can positively influence cardiovascular outcomes in women with PCOS. Dietary recommendations, regular exercise, and stress management techniques are discussed as key elements in promoting cardiovascular health. The section highlights the role of these interventions in not only managing immediate symptoms but also in preventing long-term cardiovascular complications.

7.3 Endometrial Cancer Risk

7.3.1 Unraveling the Endometrial Cancer Connection

An intriguing aspect of PCOS is its potential association with an increased risk of endometrial cancer. Chapter 7 navigates through the research linking PCOS to endometrial hyperplasia and cancer, exploring the hormonal and metabolic factors that may contribute to this elevated risk. The section emphasizes the importance of regular gynecological screenings, awareness, and individualized risk assessment for women with PCOS.

7.3.2 Preventive Strategies and Surveillance

This part of the chapter discusses preventive strategies to address the potential risk of endometrial cancer in women with PCOS. Hormonal interventions, such as oral contraceptives, are explored for their role in regulating menstrual cycles and reducing endometrial hyperplasia. The chapter also underscores the significance of maintaining a healthy weight and managing metabolic factors to further mitigate endometrial cancer risks. Regular monitoring and surveillance are presented as essential components of a comprehensive care plan for women with PCOS.

7.4 Holistic Approaches to Multifaceted Health

As Chapter 7 unfolds the intricate connections between PCOS and Type 2 diabetes, cardiovascular diseases, and endometrial cancer, it culminates in advocating for a holistic approach to health management. The chapter underscores the interconnectedness of these conditions, emphasizing the need for integrated and individualized care plans that address the unique health profile of each woman with PCOS.

7.5 Future Directions in Research and Care

To conclude, Chapter 7 provides a glimpse into the evolving landscape of PCOS research and care. Ongoing studies investigating the links between PCOS and various health conditions are highlighted. Emerging therapeutic avenues and preventive strategies are explored, offering a forward-looking perspective on the potential advancements that may shape the future of PCOS management.

By unraveling the associations between PCOS and Type 2 diabetes, cardiovascular diseases, and endometrial cancer, Chapter 7 equips readers with a comprehensive understanding of the broader health implications of PCOS. It encourages healthcare providers and individuals with

PCOS to adopt a proactive and integrated approach to care, fostering not only the management of immediate symptoms but also the prevention of long-term health risks. The chapter serves as a bridge between the realms of reproductive endocrinology and broader health management, empowering individuals with PCOS to navigate their health journey with knowledge and resilience.

CHAPTER 8

LIFESTYLE AND DIETARY GUIDELINES FOR PCOS

Polycystic Ovary Syndrome (PCOS) is a complex endocrine disorder that often necessitates a multifaceted approach to management. Chapter 8 delves into the crucial role of lifestyle and dietary modifications in mitigating PCOS symptoms and promoting overall well-being. From nutrition plans to exercise routines and weight management strategies, this chapter offers practical insights and evidence-based guidance to empower individuals with PCOS on their journey to optimal health.

8.1 Nutrition Plans

8.1.1 The Impact of Diet on PCOS Symptoms

Chapter 8 begins by elucidating the profound impact of diet on PCOS symptoms. It explores how dietary choices can influence insulin resistance, hormonal balance, and weight management—the key factors in PCOS management. By understanding the role of nutrition in PCOS, individuals can make informed decisions to optimize their dietary habits for symptom alleviation and overall health.

8.1.2 Designing a PCOS-Friendly Diet

This section provides practical guidelines for creating a PCOS-friendly diet. It explores the benefits of a low-glycemic approach, focusing on whole foods, lean proteins, and high-fiber sources. The chapter discusses the potential advantages of specific diets, such as the Mediterranean or low-carbohydrate diet, tailored to individual preferences and needs. It emphasizes the importance of moderation, variety, and mindful eating in cultivating sustainable dietary habits.

8.1.3 Nutritional Support for Hormonal Balance

Nutrition plays a pivotal role in supporting hormonal balance, particularly in the context of PCOS. Chapter 8 delves into nutrients and dietary components that may positively impact hormonal regulation. From omega-3 fatty acids to antioxidants and micronutrients like vitamin D, the section explores how specific dietary choices can contribute to hormonal equilibrium, addressing some of the root causes of PCOS symptoms.

8.2 Exercise Routines

8.2.1 The Role of Exercise in PCOS Management

Regular physical activity is a cornerstone of PCOS management, influencing insulin sensitivity, weight regulation, and overall well-being. Chapter 8 elucidates the benefits of exercise for individuals with PCOS, explaining how different types of physical activity can address specific symptoms. From aerobic exercises to strength training and flexibility routines, the chapter guides individuals in tailoring an exercise regimen that suits their preferences and lifestyle.

8.2.2 Developing a Personalized Exercise Plan

This section provides practical insights into developing a personalized exercise plan for PCOS management. It explores the frequency, intensity, and duration of exercise sessions, taking into consideration individual fitness levels and goals. The chapter also discusses the potential benefits of incorporating activities like yoga or Pilates for stress management, highlighting the holistic impact of exercise on both physical and mental well-being.

8.2.3 Overcoming Barriers to Physical Activity

Recognizing that incorporating exercise into daily life can be challenging, Chapter 8 addresses common barriers and provides strategies to overcome them. From time constraints to motivation issues, the chapter offers practical tips and motivational guidance to help individuals overcome obstacles and make physical activity an enjoyable and sustainable part of their routine.

8.3 Weight Management Strategies

8.3.1 The Interconnection of Weight and PCOS

Weight management is a critical aspect of PCOS care, influencing hormonal balance and metabolic health. Chapter 8 explores the interconnection between weight and PCOS symptoms, shedding light on how excess weight can exacerbate insulin resistance and androgen levels. It emphasizes the importance of setting realistic and achievable weight management goals for individuals with PCOS.

8.3.2 Nutrition and Exercise in Weight Management

This section integrates the earlier discussions on nutrition plans and exercise routines into a comprehensive approach to weight management for individuals with PCOS. The chapter outlines evidence-based strategies for achieving and maintaining a healthy weight, emphasizing the synergy between balanced nutrition and regular physical activity in promoting sustainable weight loss.

8.3.3 Psychological Aspects of Weight Management

Weight management is not only a physical endeavor but also involves psychological aspects. Chapter 8 addresses the emotional components of weight management, discussing strategies for cultivating a positive body image, managing stress-related eating, and fostering a healthy relationship with food. The section underscores the importance of a holistic approach that considers both the physical and emotional dimensions of weight management in PCOS.

8.4 Holistic Lifestyle Integration

8.4.1 Balancing Nutrition, Exercise, and Mental Well-being

Chapter 8 concludes by emphasizing the integration of nutrition, exercise, and mental well-being into a holistic lifestyle approach for PCOS management. It explores how these elements intersect and complement each other, fostering a synergistic effect in alleviating symptoms and improving overall health. The chapter encourages individuals with PCOS to view lifestyle modifications not as isolated interventions but as interconnected components of a comprehensive and sustainable health strategy.

8.5 Resources and Support

To empower individuals on their journey toward lifestyle and dietary changes, Chapter 8 provides a curated list of resources and support networks. From reputable nutrition guides and exercise programs to online communities and support groups, the chapter equips individuals with PCOS with the tools and connections needed to navigate and sustain their lifestyle modifications successfully.

By delving into nutrition plans, exercise routines, weight management strategies, and the integration of these elements into a holistic lifestyle, Chapter 8 serves as a comprehensive guide for individuals with PCOS seeking practical and actionable insights. It empowers them to take charge of their health through informed and personalized lifestyle choices, fostering a sense of agency and well-being in the management of this complex endocrine disorder.

CHAPTER 9

SUPPORT AND RESOURCES FOR PCOS

Polycystic Ovary Syndrome (PCOS) is not just a medical condition; it's a journey that often involves navigating challenges and seeking support. Chapter 9 delves into the various avenues of support and resources available for individuals with PCOS. From support groups and educational materials to online communities and healthcare professionals, this chapter serves as a guide to help individuals connect, learn, and thrive on their PCOS journey.

9.1 Support Groups

9.1.1 Understanding the Power of Peer Support

Support groups play a crucial role in fostering a sense of community and understanding among individuals with

PCOS. Chapter 9 begins by exploring the importance of peer support in navigating the complexities of PCOS. It delves into how sharing experiences, challenges, and triumphs with others facing similar situations can provide validation, encouragement, and a sense of camaraderie.

9.1.2 Joining Local and Online Support Groups

This section offers practical advice on how individuals with PCOS can find and join local and online support groups. From community organizations to virtual forums, the chapter provides insights into where individuals can connect with others who share their experiences. It also discusses the benefits of attending in-person support group meetings and participating in online discussions, highlighting the diverse opportunities for building a supportive network.

9.1.3 Support for Specific PCOS Phenotypes

Recognizing the heterogeneity of PCOS presentations, this part of the chapter explores the availability of support groups tailored to specific PCOS phenotypes. Whether it's lean PCOS, classic PCOS, or postmenopausal PCOS, individuals can find specialized groups that address their unique challenges and provide targeted support.

9.2 Educational Materials

9.2.1 Empowering Through Knowledge

Education is a powerful tool for empowering individuals with PCOS to understand their condition and make informed decisions. Chapter 9 discusses the importance of reliable educational materials in providing comprehensive information about PCOS, its symptoms, and available management strategies. It emphasizes the role of healthcare providers, reputable websites, and educational resources in offering accurate and up-to-date information.

9.2.2 Recommended Reading and Resources

To facilitate learning, this section provides a curated list of recommended reading and resources on PCOS. From authoritative books and academic publications to trustworthy online platforms, the chapter guides individuals toward reputable sources that can enhance their understanding of PCOS and its multifaceted aspects.

9.3 Online Communities

9.3.1 Connecting Virtually

In the digital age, online communities have become invaluable spaces for individuals to connect, share, and seek advice. Chapter 9 explores the world of online communities dedicated to PCOS, highlighting the benefits of joining forums, social media groups, and interactive platforms. It discusses how these virtual spaces foster a sense of belonging and enable individuals to seek and provide support in real-time.

9.3.2 Navigating Online Communities Safely

While online communities offer tremendous support, it's essential to navigate them safely. This part of the chapter provides practical tips for engaging in online discussions responsibly, including protecting privacy, verifying information, and maintaining a positive and constructive online presence. It underscores the importance of creating a supportive online environment for everyone involved.

9.4 Healthcare Professionals

9.4.1 Building a Collaborative Relationship

Healthcare professionals play a pivotal role in the PCOS journey. Chapter 9 explores the significance of establishing a collaborative relationship with healthcare providers. It discusses the importance of open communication, regular check-ups, and proactive discussions about treatment plans, ensuring that individuals with PCOS feel heard and actively involved in their care.

9.4.2 Choosing the Right Healthcare Team

Not all healthcare professionals have the same level of expertise in PCOS management. This section guides individuals in selecting a healthcare team that specializes in reproductive endocrinology, gynecology, or endocrinology. It emphasizes the importance of finding professionals who understand the unique aspects of PCOS and can tailor treatment plans to individual needs.

9.5 Advocacy and Awareness

9.5.1 Empowering Through Advocacy

Advocacy is a powerful tool for effecting change and raising awareness about PCOS. Chapter 9 discusses the role of advocacy in empowering individuals and communities to drive policy changes, improve healthcare access, and foster greater understanding of PCOS. It explores how individuals can become advocates for themselves and the broader PCOS community.

9.5.2 Participating in Awareness Campaigns

To encourage active participation, this part of the chapter provides information on various PCOS awareness campaigns and initiatives. Whether it's PCOS Awareness Month or specific advocacy events, individuals can contribute to raising awareness by sharing their stories, engaging with campaigns, and participating in community events.

9.6 Coping Strategies and Self-Care

9.6.1 Nurturing Mental and Emotional Well-being

Living with PCOS involves not only physical challenges but also mental and emotional aspects. Chapter 9 explores coping strategies and self-care practices that can enhance mental and emotional well-being. From mindfulness techniques to creative outlets and self-compassion exercises, the chapter provides a toolkit for individuals to navigate the emotional dimensions of their PCOS journey.

9.6.2 Balancing Self-Care with Advocacy
Recognizing the interconnected nature of self-care and advocacy, this section discusses how individuals can strike a balance between taking care of themselves and contributing to the greater PCOS community. It emphasizes the importance of self-compassion and self-advocacy in fostering resilience and creating a positive impact on both personal and collective well-being.

9.7 Building Resilience for the PCOS Journey

9.7.1 Embracing Resilience
Chapter 9 concludes by focusing on the concept of resilience in the context of the PCOS journey. It explores how resilience, the ability to bounce back from challenges, can be cultivated through support networks, education, self-care, and advocacy. The chapter leaves readers with

empowering insights on building resilience and thriving on their unique PCOS journey.

By addressing support groups, educational materials, online communities, healthcare professionals, advocacy, coping strategies, and resilience, Chapter 9 serves as a comprehensive guide to the support and resources available for individuals with PCOS. It empowers them to connect with others, stay informed, seek professional guidance, and foster resilience, ultimately enhancing their ability to navigate the complexities of living with PCOS.

CHAPTER 10

FUTURE DIRECTIONS IN PCOS RESEARCH

Polycystic Ovary Syndrome (PCOS) is a dynamic field of study, and ongoing research continually unveils new insights into its causes, manifestations, and potential treatment approaches. Chapter 10 delves into the exciting realm of future directions in PCOS research, exploring emerging areas of study, innovative therapies, and potential breakthroughs that hold promise for improving the understanding and management of this complex endocrine disorder.

10.1 Ongoing Studies

10.1.1 Investigating Genetic and Environmental Factors
Genetic and environmental factors contribute significantly to the development of PCOS, and ongoing studies aim to

unravel the intricate interplay between these elements. Chapter 10 explores how researchers are delving into the genomic landscape to identify specific genes associated with PCOS susceptibility. Additionally, it discusses studies investigating the impact of environmental factors such as diet, lifestyle, and exposure to endocrine-disrupting chemicals on the development and progression of PCOS.

10.1.2 Longitudinal Studies on PCOS Phenotypes

Recognizing the heterogeneity of PCOS presentations, researchers are increasingly turning to longitudinal studies to track the progression of different PCOS phenotypes over time. This section delves into the significance of understanding how PCOS evolves throughout a woman's life, providing insights into potential predictors of long-term complications and tailoring interventions to specific phenotypic expressions.

10.2 Potential Breakthroughs

10.2.1 Advancements in Hormonal Therapies

The quest for more targeted and effective hormonal therapies for PCOS is a focal point of current research.

Chapter 10 explores potential breakthroughs in hormonal interventions, such as the development of novel anti-androgen medications with enhanced specificity and reduced side effects. It also delves into studies investigating the optimal formulation and delivery methods for hormonal treatments to maximize efficacy and minimize adverse reactions.

10.2.2 Personalized Medicine and Treatment Plans

The era of personalized medicine is influencing PCOS research, aiming to tailor treatment plans based on individual characteristics, genetics, and phenotypic variations. This section explores how advancements in genetic testing, biomarker identification, and artificial intelligence are paving the way for more precise and personalized approaches to PCOS management. The chapter discusses the potential impact of personalized medicine in optimizing treatment outcomes and minimizing side effects.

10.3 Lifestyle Interventions and Digital Health

10.3.1 Integrating Technology for Lifestyle Management

The integration of technology into lifestyle interventions is a burgeoning area of research in PCOS. Chapter 10 explores studies investigating the effectiveness of digital health platforms, mobile applications, and wearable devices in supporting individuals with PCOS in their journey towards improved nutrition, regular exercise, and stress management. It discusses how these tools can enhance adherence, provide real-time feedback, and foster long-term behavior change.

10.3.2 Virtual Health Coaching and Telemedicine

Virtual health coaching and telemedicine are emerging as potential game-changers in PCOS care. This section delves into studies exploring the efficacy of virtual health coaching programs, where individuals receive personalized guidance and support remotely. It also discusses the role of telemedicine in expanding access to specialized care, allowing individuals to consult with PCOS experts regardless of geographical barriers.

10.4 Fertility Advancements

10.4.1 Innovations in Assisted Reproductive Technologies

Advancements in assisted reproductive technologies (ART) are reshaping the landscape of fertility interventions for women with PCOS. Chapter 10 explores studies investigating innovative approaches within ART, such as improvements in in vitro fertilization (IVF) protocols, the utilization of artificial intelligence in embryo selection, and the potential role of uterine microbiota in implantation success. The section discusses how these advancements may enhance the chances of successful pregnancies for individuals with PCOS.

10.4.2 Preservation of Ovarian Function

Preserving ovarian function is a key consideration for women with PCOS, particularly those facing fertility challenges. This part of the chapter explores research on ovarian tissue cryopreservation and other emerging techniques aimed at preserving fertility potential. It discusses the potential implications of these advancements for women with PCOS who may consider delaying childbearing for personal or medical reasons.

10.5 Addressing Metabolic and Cardiovascular Risks

10.5.1 Targeting Insulin Resistance with Precision

Given the central role of insulin resistance in PCOS, researchers are exploring precision medicine approaches to target insulin resistance more effectively. Chapter 10 delves into studies investigating novel insulin-sensitizing agents, individualized dietary recommendations based on metabolic profiles, and the integration of gut microbiota research to modulate metabolic outcomes. It explores how these advancements may lead to more targeted and tailored interventions for individuals with PCOS at risk of metabolic complications.

10.5.2 Cardiovascular Risk Prediction Models

Predicting cardiovascular risk in women with PCOS is a complex task, considering the multifactorial nature of cardiovascular complications. This section explores studies developing and validating predictive models that incorporate various risk factors specific to PCOS. It discusses how these models may enhance risk stratification, allowing for earlier interventions and personalized cardiovascular care for individuals with PCOS.

10.6 Psychosocial and Mental Health Considerations

10.6.1 Integrating Mental Health Support

Recognizing the impact of PCOS on mental health, researchers are focusing on integrated approaches that address both physical and psychological well-being. Chapter 10 explores studies evaluating the effectiveness of integrated mental health support within PCOS care, ranging from counseling and psychotherapy to mindfulness-based interventions. It discusses how such approaches may contribute to a more comprehensive and holistic model of PCOS management.

10.6.2 Online Mental Health Platforms

The utilization of online mental health platforms and telepsychiatry services is gaining traction in PCOS research. This section delves into studies examining the feasibility and efficacy of virtual mental health support for individuals with PCOS. It discusses how online platforms may enhance accessibility, reduce stigma, and provide tailored mental health interventions for those navigating the emotional complexities of PCOS.

10.7 Patient-Researcher Collaboration

10.7.1 Shaping Research Priorities Together

An emerging trend in PCOS research involves fostering collaboration between researchers and individuals with PCOS. Chapter 10 explores studies that prioritize patient perspectives, involving individuals with PCOS in the research process from study design to implementation. It discusses how such collaborative approaches can ensure that research aligns with the priorities and needs of the PCOS community, leading to more meaningful and patient-centered outcomes.

10.7.2 Citizen Science Initiatives

Citizen science initiatives are empowering individuals with PCOS to actively participate in research. This part of the chapter explores studies leveraging citizen science to collect data, share experiences, and contribute to scientific advancements in PCOS. It discusses how these initiatives democratize research, making it more inclusive and reflective of the diverse experiences within the PCOS community.

10.8 Ethical Considerations and Future Challenges

10.8.1 Ethical Dimensions of PCOS Research

As PCOS research evolves, ethical considerations become paramount. Chapter 10 explores the ethical dimensions of PCOS research, from ensuring informed consent and data privacy to addressing disparities in research representation. It discusses how researchers and the PCOS community can collaborate to navigate ethical challenges and foster a research environment grounded in transparency and respect.

10.8.2 Overcoming Research Gaps and Disparities

Despite advancements, research gaps and disparities persist in PCOS studies. This section discusses ongoing challenges, such as limited representation of diverse populations, gaps in understanding specific PCOS phenotypes, and the need for more long-term studies. It explores strategies to address these challenges and foster an inclusive and comprehensive research landscape.

10.9 Shaping the Future of PCOS Care

10.9.1 From Bench to Bedside

The translation of research findings into tangible improvements in PCOS care is the ultimate goal. Chapter 10 explores how research endeavors contribute to the evolution of PCOS care—from innovative therapies to personalized treatment plans. It emphasizes the importance of bridging the gap between research discoveries and clinical applications to ensure that individuals with PCOS benefit from the latest advancements.

10.9.2 Empowering Individuals Through Research

This section underscores the empowering role of research in the lives of individuals with PCOS. It discusses how being informed about ongoing research, participating in studies, and contributing to the shaping of research priorities can empower individuals to actively engage with their healthcare journey. The chapter encourages a collaborative approach where individuals with PCOS become partners in research, driving the evolution of PCOS care.

Chapter 10 serves as a beacon into the future of PCOS research, highlighting the exciting avenues that researchers are exploring to deepen our understanding and improve the management of this complex syndrome. It underscores the dynamic nature of PCOS research, with ongoing studies shaping a future where individuals with PCOS can benefit from more targeted, personalized, and holistic approaches to their care.

CHAPTER 11

CONCLUSION - EMPOWERING INDIVIDUALS WITH PCOS

The journey through Polycystic Ovary Syndrome (PCOS) has been an exploration of complexities, challenges, and opportunities. As we conclude this comprehensive guide, Chapter 11 serves as a synthesis of key points, an empowerment manifesto for individuals with PCOS, and a glance into the future of PCOS care.

11.1 Recapitulation of Key Points

The preceding chapters have intricately unraveled the multifaceted nature of PCOS, from its pathophysiology and clinical manifestations to diagnostic approaches, management strategies, and the psychosocial dimensions that individuals grapple with. Key points deserving recapitulation include the hormonal imbalances involving elevated androgens and insulin resistance, the challenges posed by anovulation and irregular menstrual cycles, and the association of PCOS with various health conditions such as diabetes, cardiovascular risks, and endometrial cancer.

Furthermore, the chapters have navigated through lifestyle and dietary considerations, shedding light on the pivotal role of nutrition, exercise, and weight management in PCOS management. Support and resources have been explored extensively, emphasizing the significance of peer support, educational materials, online communities, and collaborative relationships with healthcare professionals. The future directions in PCOS research have been outlined, highlighting ongoing studies, potential breakthroughs, and the evolving landscape of personalized and holistic care.

11.2 Empowering Individuals with PCOS

Empowerment lies at the heart of navigating life with PCOS. Chapter 11 aims to instill a sense of empowerment in individuals with PCOS by reinforcing the understanding that knowledge is a powerful tool. Armed with a comprehensive understanding of their condition, individuals can actively engage with their healthcare journey, make informed decisions, and advocate for their needs.

11.2.1 Knowledge as a Catalyst for Self-Advocacy

Being informed about PCOS empowers individuals to become advocates for themselves. From understanding the intricacies of hormonal imbalances to grasping the impact of lifestyle choices, knowledge serves as a catalyst for self-advocacy. Informed individuals are better equipped to communicate with healthcare professionals, actively participate in treatment decisions, and shape their healthcare journey according to their unique needs.

11.2.2 Navigating Lifestyle Changes with Confidence

The lifestyle and dietary guidelines provided in this guide are not rigid prescriptions but tools for individuals to tailor to their preferences and needs. Empowerment in the context of PCOS involves navigating lifestyle changes with confidence. Whether it's adopting a PCOS-friendly diet, engaging in regular exercise, or managing weight, individuals are encouraged to embrace these changes as positive steps towards holistic well-being.

11.2.3 Building a Support Network

Recognizing the importance of peer support and community, empowerment in Chapter 11 extends to building a robust support network. Engaging with support groups, connecting with others facing similar challenges, and participating in online communities contribute to a sense of belonging. Sharing experiences, triumphs, and setbacks fosters a supportive environment where individuals feel understood and encouraged on their PCOS journey.

11.2.4 Collaborating with Healthcare Professionals

Empowerment also involves fostering collaborative relationships with healthcare professionals. Chapter 11 reinforces the idea that individuals should actively engage with their healthcare team, communicate openly about their concerns, and work collaboratively to tailor treatment plans. The guide advocates for selecting healthcare professionals with expertise in PCOS, ensuring that individuals receive specialized and informed care.

11.2.5 Balancing Self-Care with Advocacy

A delicate balance between self-care and advocacy is crucial for individuals with PCOS. Chapter 11 encourages individuals to prioritize their mental and emotional well-being, engage in coping strategies, and nurture resilience. Simultaneously, it emphasizes the potential for individuals to contribute to the broader PCOS community through advocacy, awareness campaigns, and participation in research initiatives.

11.3 Future Perspectives in PCOS Care

The concluding chapter peeks into the future of PCOS care, recognizing the dynamic nature of research and healthcare advancements. From ongoing studies investigating genetic and environmental factors to potential breakthroughs in hormonal therapies and personalized medicine, the future holds promise for more targeted and individualized approaches to PCOS management.

11.3.1 Patient-Researcher Collaboration

A noteworthy aspect of the future of PCOS care is the collaboration between patients and researchers. Chapter 11 underscores the importance of patient perspectives in shaping research priorities and outcomes. Initiatives such as citizen science and participatory research emphasize the democratization of research, ensuring that the diverse experiences within the PCOS community contribute to scientific advancements.

13.3.2 Ethical Considerations and Inclusivity

As PCOS research evolves, ethical considerations take center stage. The guide emphasizes the importance of addressing ethical dimensions, ensuring informed consent, protecting data privacy, and overcoming disparities in research representation. An inclusive and ethical approach to PCOS research is pivotal for fostering transparency, trust, and respect within the research community.

11.3.3 Bridging the Gap between Research and Clinical Practice

The translation of research findings into tangible improvements in clinical practice is a key theme in Chapter

11. From hormonal therapies and lifestyle interventions to fertility advancements and cardiovascular risk prediction models, the future of PCOS care involves bridging the gap between research discoveries and their application in real-world healthcare settings.

Conclusion

In conclusion, Chapter 11 encapsulates the essence of empowerment for individuals with PCOS. Through knowledge, self-advocacy, lifestyle changes, support networks, collaboration with healthcare professionals, and a glimpse into the future of PCOS care, this guide aims to equip individuals with the tools they need to navigate their unique PCOS journey with resilience, confidence, and a sense of empowerment. As the landscape of PCOS care evolves, individuals are encouraged to stay informed, actively engage in their healthcare, and contribute to the collective empowerment of the PCOS community.

Made in the USA
Thornton, CO
05/30/24 11:01:08

f2d69862-2c8f-4c29-ba5c-668187a1f595R01